W9-BGR-643

"ANIMALS, VEGETABLES AND MINERALS — FROM A TO Z *travels through the complex world of nutrition in such an interesting way that kids and adults will be drawn in.*

—Dr. Jeffrey Friedman, D.O. Family Practice, South Daytona, FL

"Teacher-terrific and author Sallie O'Donnell has crafted a delightful and fun book to inspire kids to get on the right track to healthy eating."

— Michael Murphy, Orlando Sentinel op-ed editor

"I read this book to my 4 year-old granddaughter and she keeps telling me about the quail who never overeats and the cougar building speed with calcium. Kids will love the book and grandparents will love talking to the kids about it."

— William D.A. Hill, weekly columnist for the Daily News Journal, New Smyrna Beach, FL, retired editor, film writer, reporter and magazine writer

"ANIMALS, VEGETABLES AND MINERALS — FROM A TO Z *makes eating your vegetables an A to Z adventure!"*

— Jennifer Elin Cole, co-author "I Love You All The Time" and mother of three, Atlanta, GA

"This book provides a colorful, fun, creative way to introduce nutritional concepts to children. A must for any medical facility or institution that holds the interests of children's health and wellness at heart."

— Dr. Hatha Gbedawo, Naturopathic Physician, Seattle, WA

"ANIMALS, VEGETABLES AND MINERALS — FROM A TO Z *has all the qualities of becoming a classic. Kids will love it! Parents will love reading it to them."*

— Laura Parente, assistant principal , Intermediate School 126, Queens, New York

"Sallie O'Donnell needs to be applauded for her verses which teach healthy eating for a generation in need. She is able to weave nutritional concepts into messages that are lasting and timely for everyone!"
— Jeffrey Whitridge, RD LD/N, Clinical Dietitian/Nutritionist, Asheville, NC

"There is a Dr. Seuss quality to this book. The humorous verses convey important information in an entertaining and educational fashion and address the need to teach healthy nutritional habits early on in life."
— Dr. Steven R. Sabat, Professor of Psychology,
Georgetown University, Washington, DC

*"*ANIMALS, VEGETABLES AND MINERALS — FROM A TO Z *is not only informative, it is a delight to read."*
— Howard L. Hurwitz, Ph. D., retired principal,
Jamaica, New York

*"*ANIMALS, VEGETABLES AND MINERALS — FROM A TO Z *uses clever, alliterative rhymes combined with unique illustrations to develop language skills while promoting good nutrition. This book will hold the interest of both adult readers and young listeners."*
— Jean McMullan, assistant principal (retired),
English instruction, New York City Public Schools

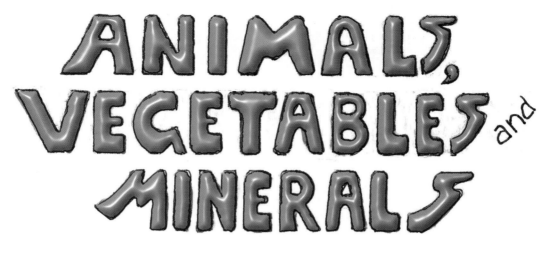

ANIMALS, VEGETABLES and MINERALS

from A to Z

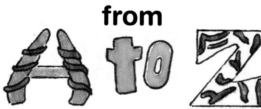

Story by Sallie O'Donnell

Illustrations by Alea Plumley

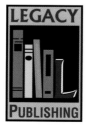

LEGACY PUBLISHING SERVICES

602 N. Wymore Road Winter Park, Florida 32789

www.LegacyPublishingServices.com

Published by:
LEGACY PUBLISHING SERVICES
602 N. Wymore Road
Winter Park, Florida 32789
www.legacypublishingservices.com

Copyright © 2005 by Sallie M. O'Donnell
ISBN 0-9764982-5-1
Cover and interior illustrations by Alea Plumley

For comments to the author, scheduling interviews or speaking engagements, contact through the *authors'* page at www.legacypublishingservices.com.

Printed in S. Korea

All rights reserved. Written permission must be secured from the publisher to use or reproduce any part of this book, except for brief critical reviews or articles.

In loving memory of my parents

Ida and Ben Rubin

Where it all began………………

Acknowledgements

First to my family: To my daughter, Bonnie, and my son, Ben, for all the joy you have brought to me from day one; your love, support and encouragement keep me going and persevering every day. To their spouses, Don and Sue, for bringing great love, companionship and happiness to my "kids" and always being there for me as well. To my 3 grandchildren of whom I am extraordinarily proud. I love you all. To my beloved cousin, Mindy, for her constant faith in me through the years. You're the sister I never had. To my husband, John, a.k.a. Mr. Wonderful, thanks honey for sticking by me through stormy seas and strong winds. Without you there would be no book.

To the R.E.A.D. book club for their friendship and support. To Eesha for the introduction, Florence, most patient photographer, for listening, Mara for the connection, BJ for the generous offer, H.G., Dr. Jeff and Dr. Pam — you know why. To Alea Plumley, artist extraordinaire, who illustrated, enhanced and brought spirit and life to my verses. And, to the thousands of students who entered my classroom over my 33 year career, thanks for all the lessons I learned from you and for giving my life purpose and meaning.

Sallie M. O'Donnell

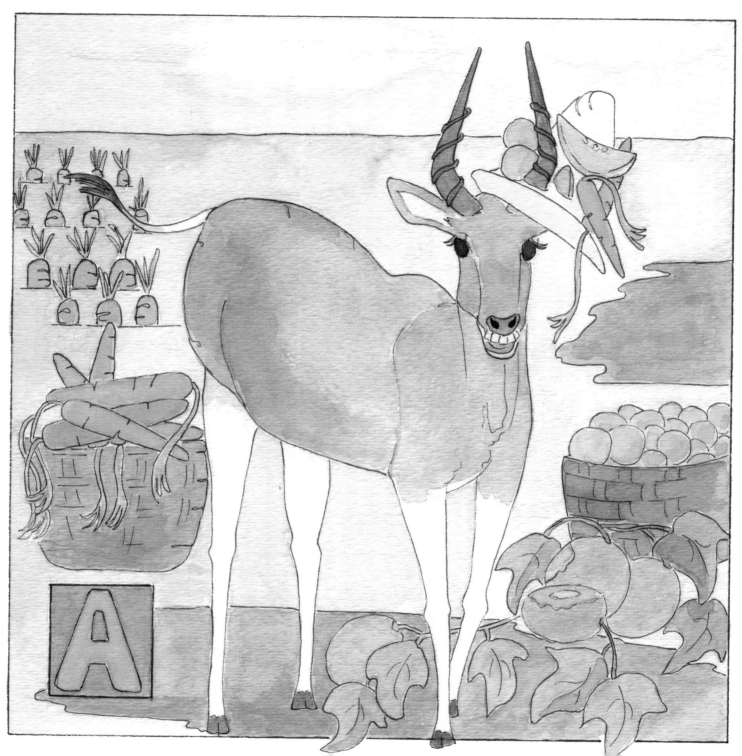

"I get vitamin A," says
  the long-legged antelope

"From a carrot or peach
  or a very nice cantaloupe.

It's good for my skin,
  and it helps fight infection

And gives my teeth and
  bones added protection."

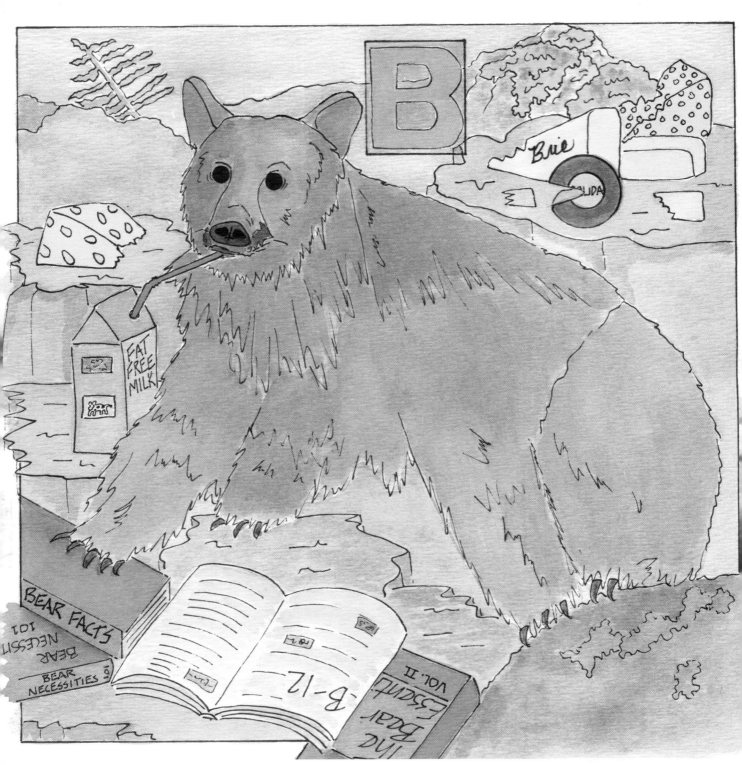

Into large reference books
the bear need not delve,

To uncover the bare facts
about vitamin B-12.

A major blood builder
and aid to new growth,

He stocks dairy products
to assure he gets both.

BEARLY

Grizzly Facts of B-12

B.E. Grizzly

Bear All

DARE to CARE:
BE A HEALTHY BEAR

YOGI'S Diet Book

CHUBBY CUBBIES

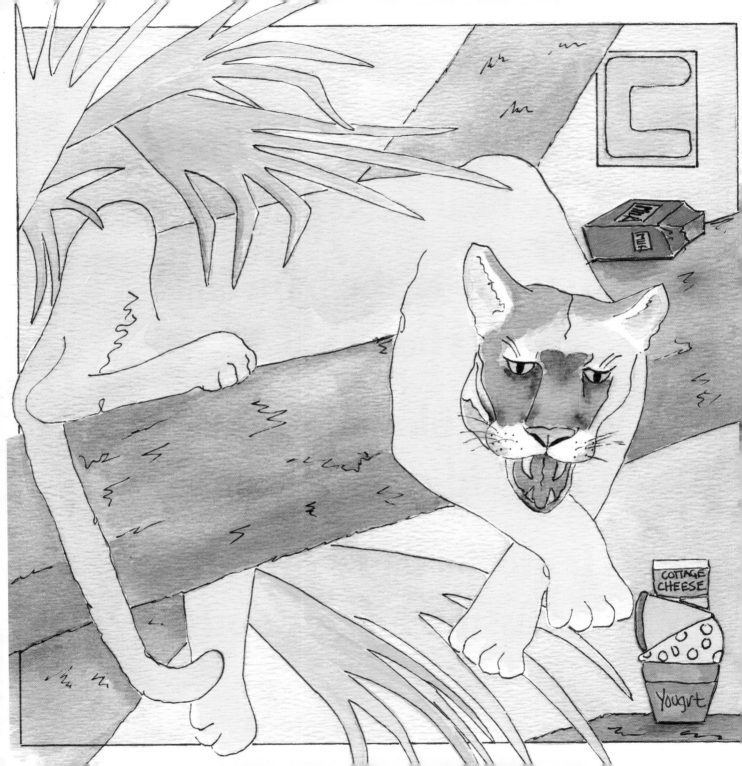

Calcium for the cougar
who's fast on the curves,

Is ideal for clotting
and calming its nerves.

It also builds strong bones
and teeth that look neat

And is found in milk products
and whole grains like wheat.

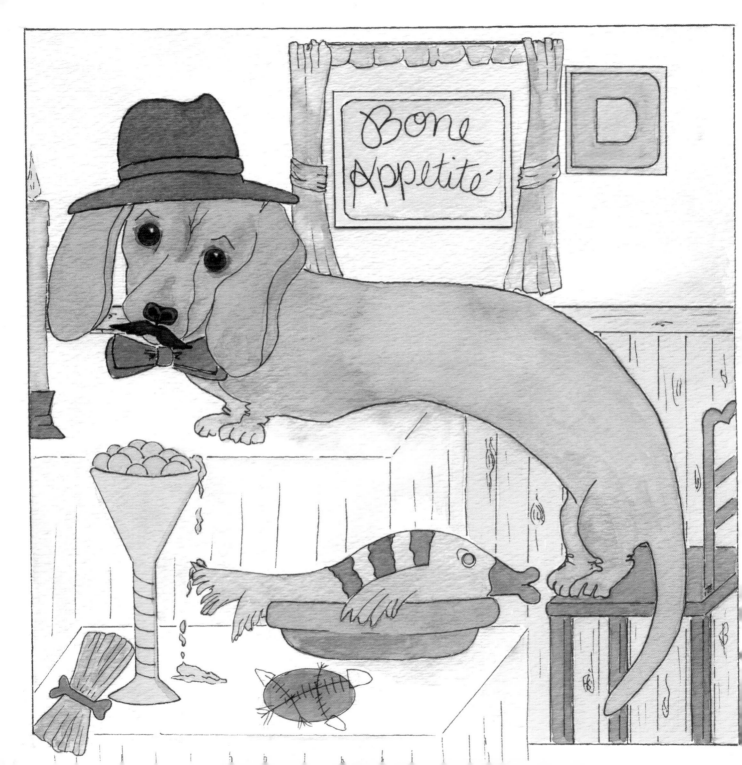

"D is a vitamin
    perfect for me."

Drawls the debonair dachshund,
    "That's why I agree

To eat egg yolks and fish
    to keep my muscles strong

And build up my bones
    some of which are quite long."

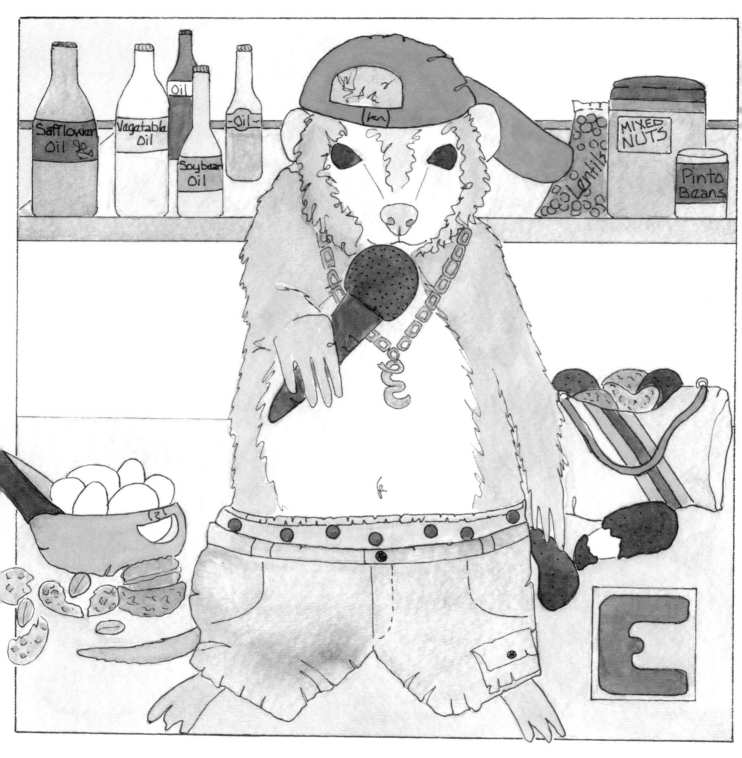

"Welcome," raps the ermine warmly,
"take a tip from me.

Vegetable, soybean, and safflower
oils are rich in vitamin E.

So are eggs, legumes and
nuts minus shells.

These will help provide
long life to red blood cells."

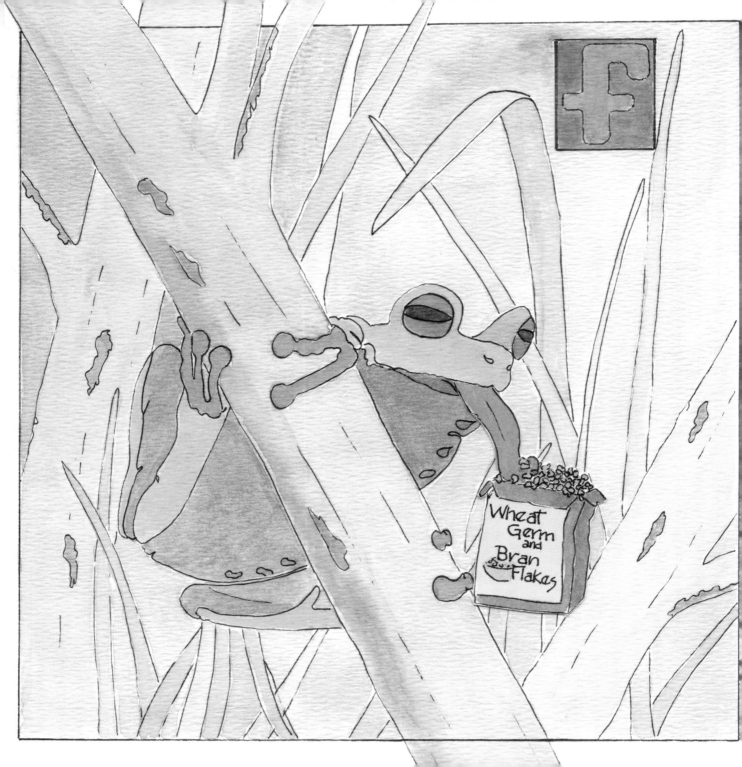

"Fiber's my way,"
   the funky frog croaks

"Of cleaning my system
   — take my word folks.

Fast foods and bleached flour
   all processed by man

Will not do the job like
   raw wheat germ and bran."

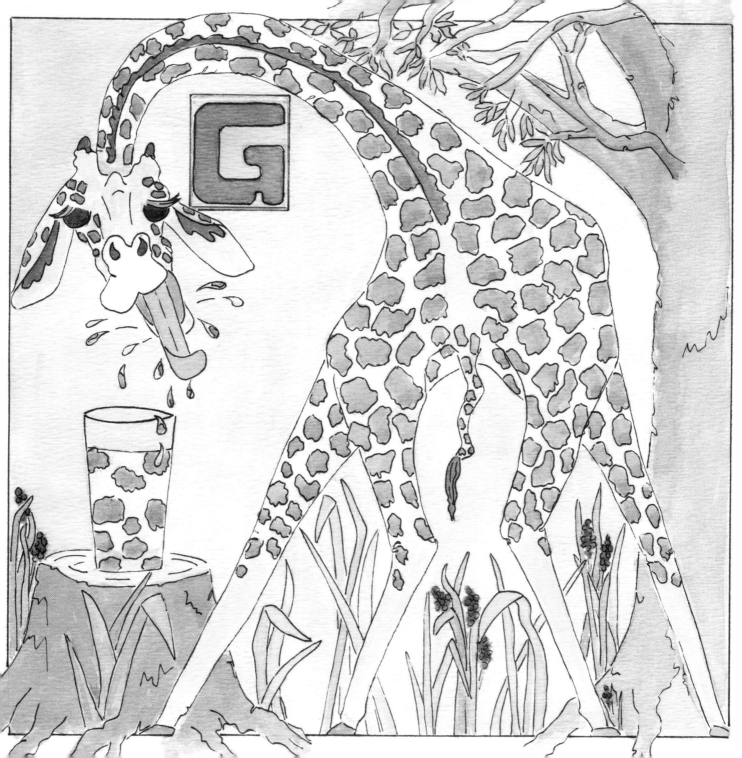

The graceful giraffe glances
down feeling placid

From the effects of
gamma linolenic acid

Which he gets from his
mommy's milk that doesn't spoil

Also found in evening
primrose — that's oil!

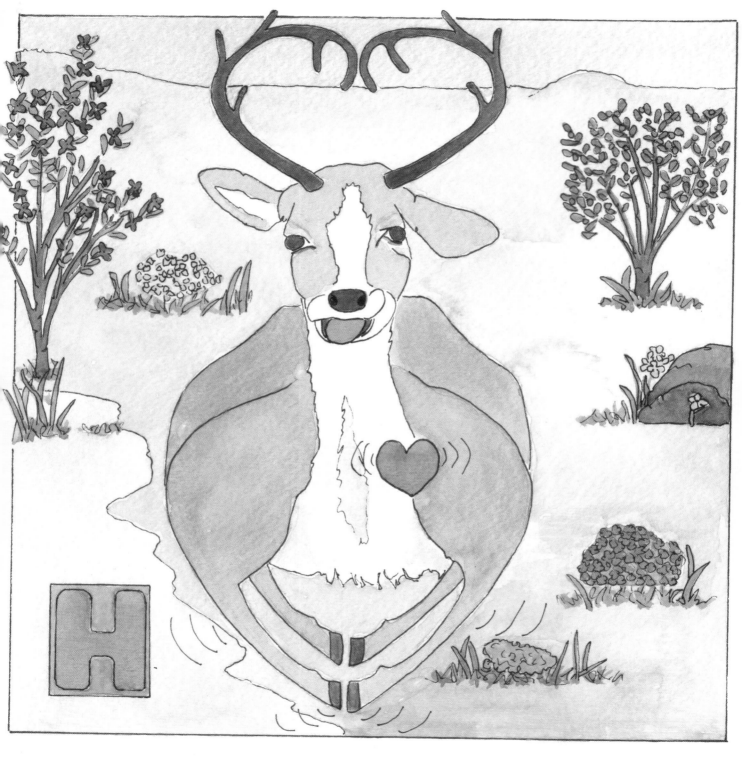

Because he thinks sitting
around is all wrong

The hart is an animal
healthy and strong

When out in the fields
he is romping and jumping

For he knows exercise will
keep his heart pumping.

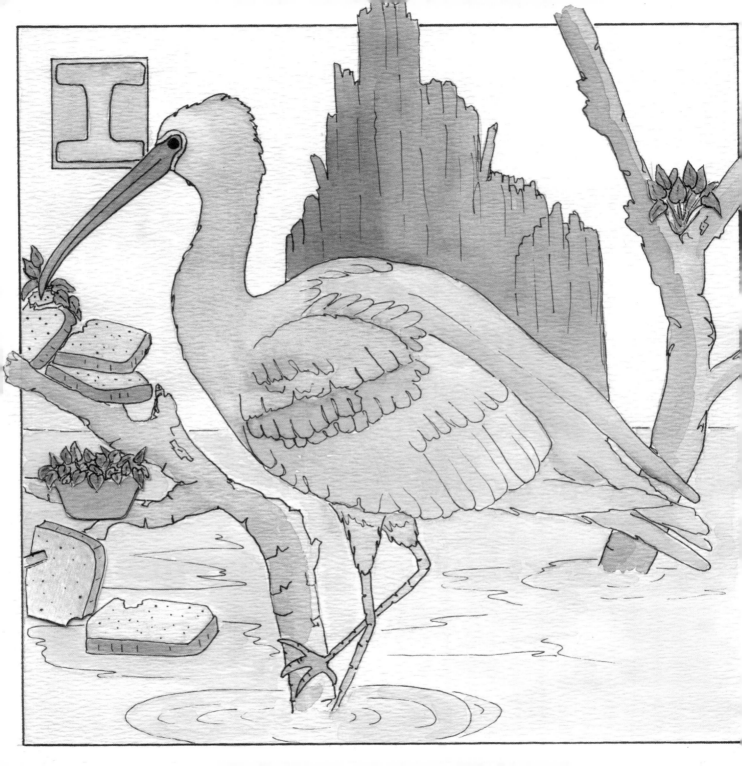

Why the ibis picks iron
is easy to guess

'Cause it helps build up blood
and resistance to stress.

Whole grain breads and spinach
have an ample supply

Of this mineral whose
import one cannot deny.

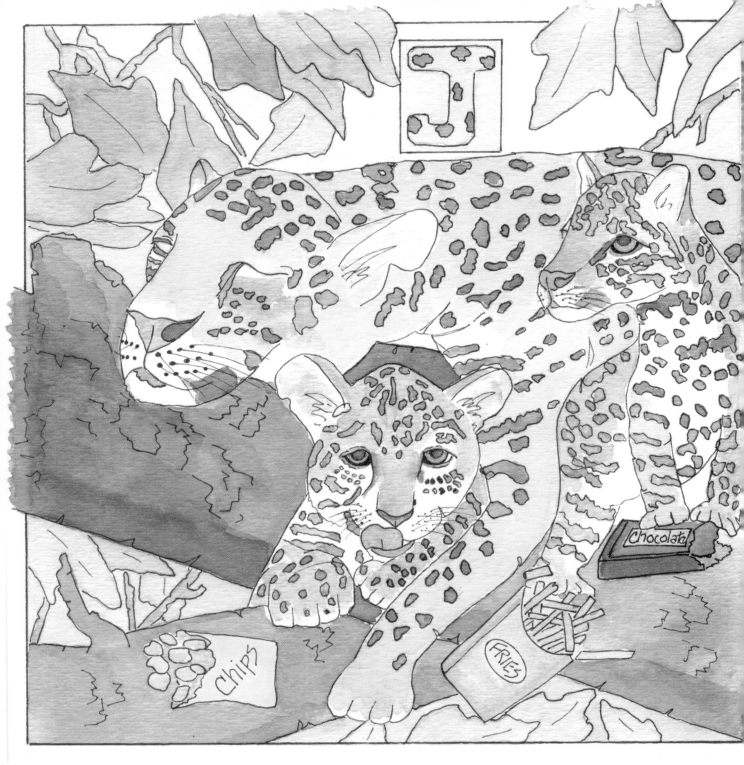

The jovial jaguar
nestles her brood

As she warns against eating
unhealthy junk food.

"It's bad for your teeth and
no good for your system.

Pay careful attention to
these words of wisdom."

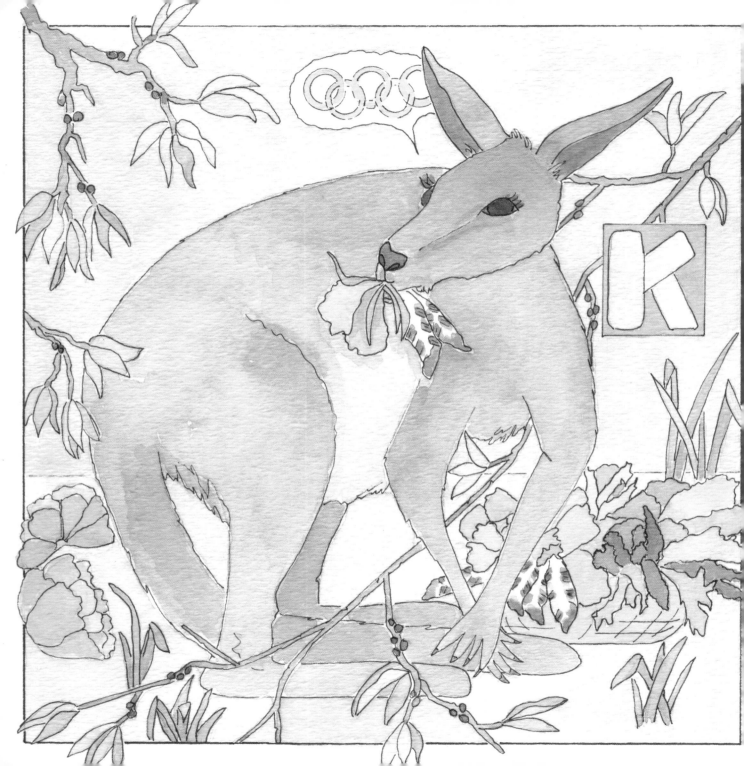

Vitamin K is the choice
of the spry kangaroo

Chewing leafy green vegetables
and alfalfa too.

She plans a long life filled
with good health and vigor

And will hop in the Olympics
when she gets a bit bigger.

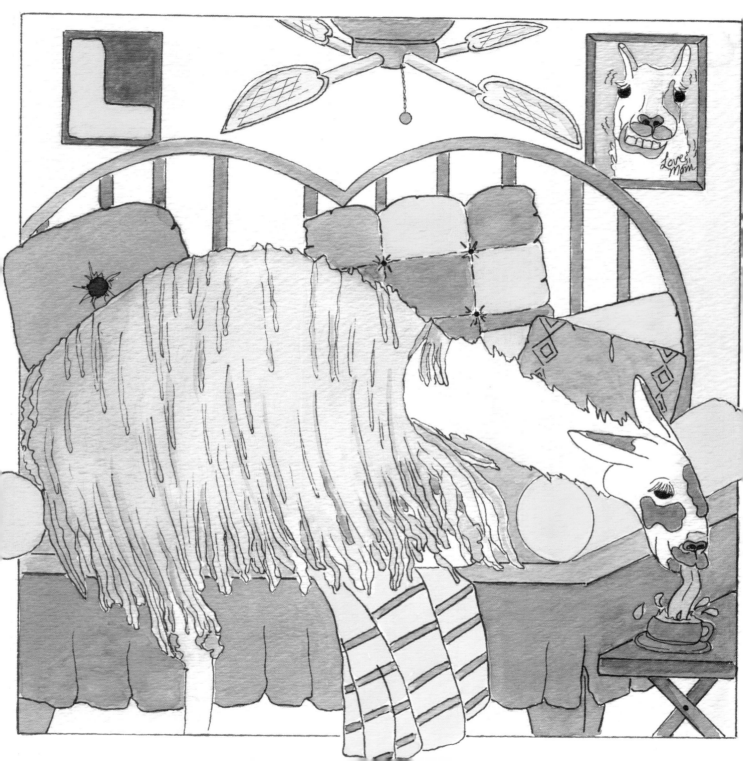

The languorous llama
  laps soy bean oil

Rich in lecithin,
  which is a natural foil

'Gainst building up deposits
  of fat in the liver.

The thought of which makes
  her whole family quiver.

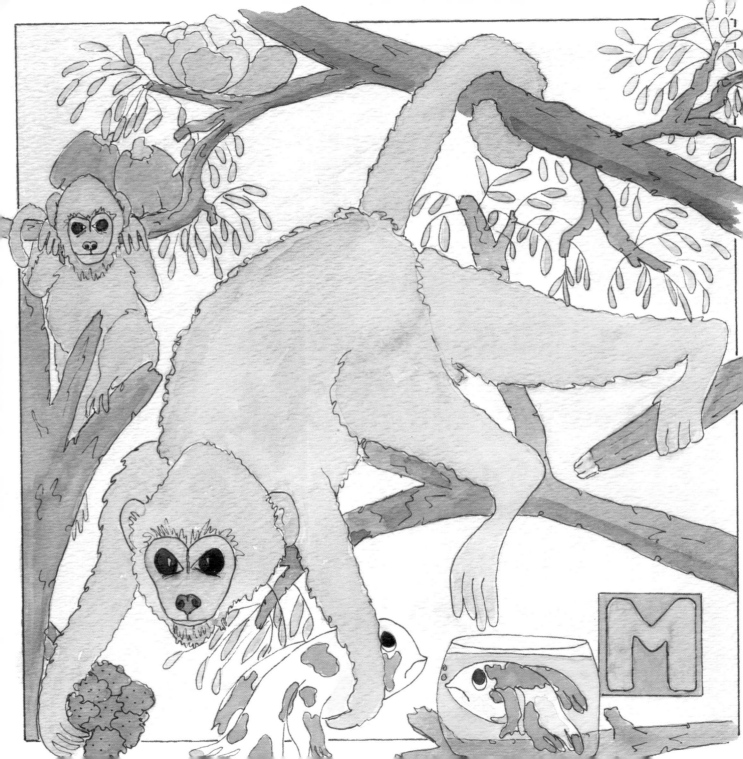

Monkeys have a calm life
although they stay busy,

They swing upside down
and never get dizzy.

Consuming much fish, meat
and veggies quite green

All containing magnesium
which keeps them serene.

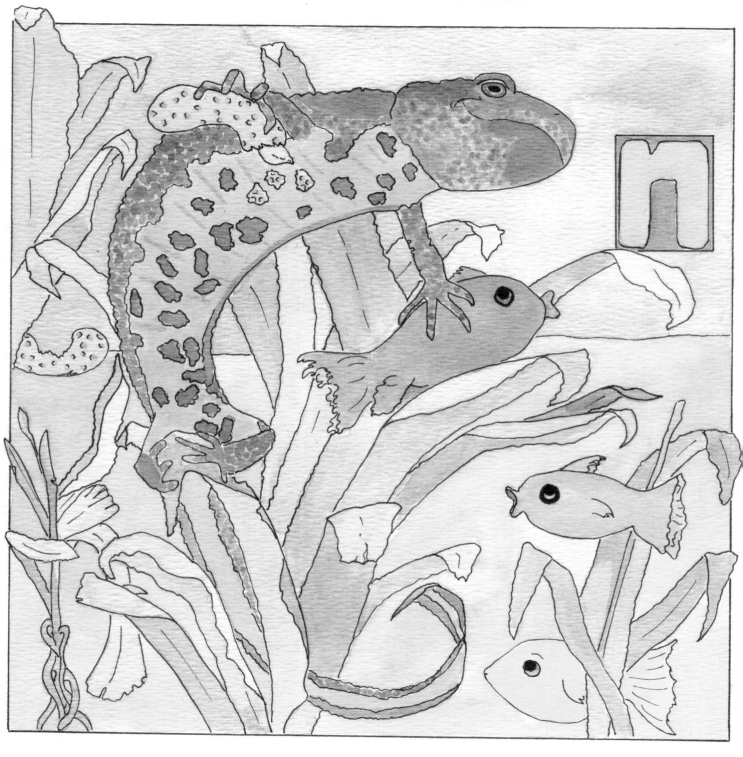

Niacin, in other words,
vitamin B-3

Found in peanuts and poultry
and fish from the sea

Keeps the digestive system
tip-top for the newt

So tiny there's no doubt
that she is trés cute.

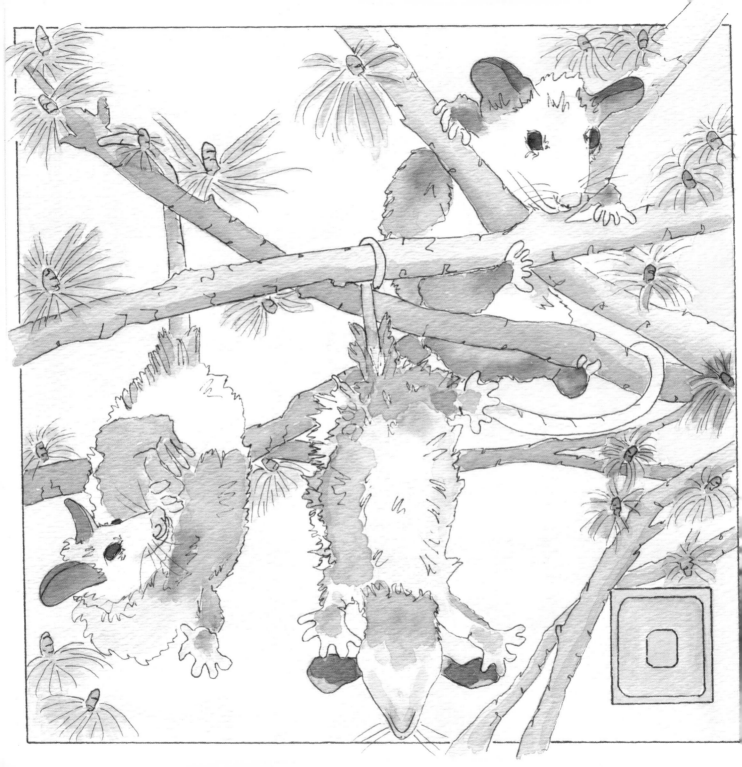

Swinging and hanging
around with the guys

The opossum gets oodles
of great exercise

And fresh oxygen a must
in any season

That's what gives this
rhyme a good reason.

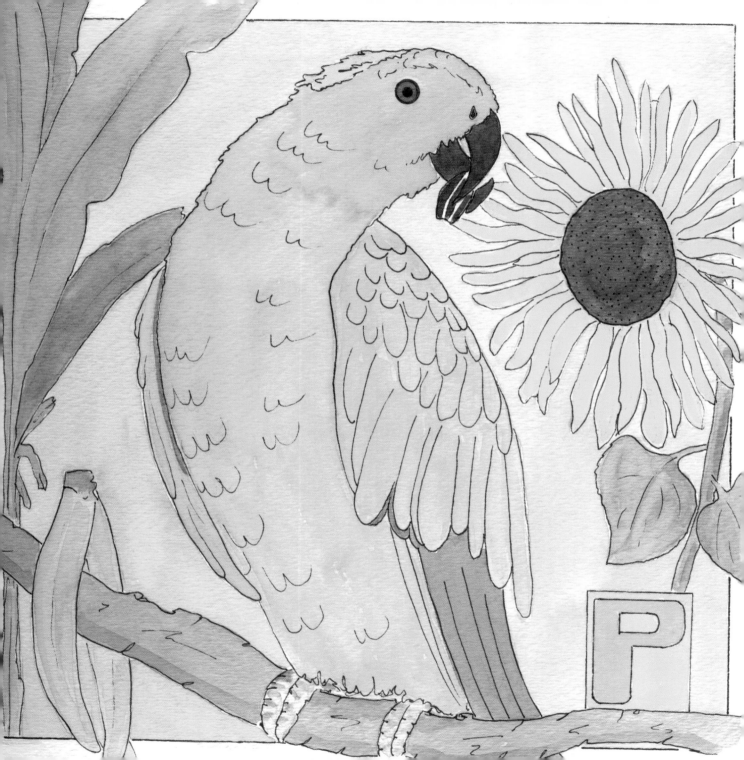

"Potassium," pipes the parrot
munching sunflower seeds,

"Is essential for maintaining
a lot of the needs

Of my muscles and nerves.
So at all of my meals

I dine on bananas
and potatoes with peels."

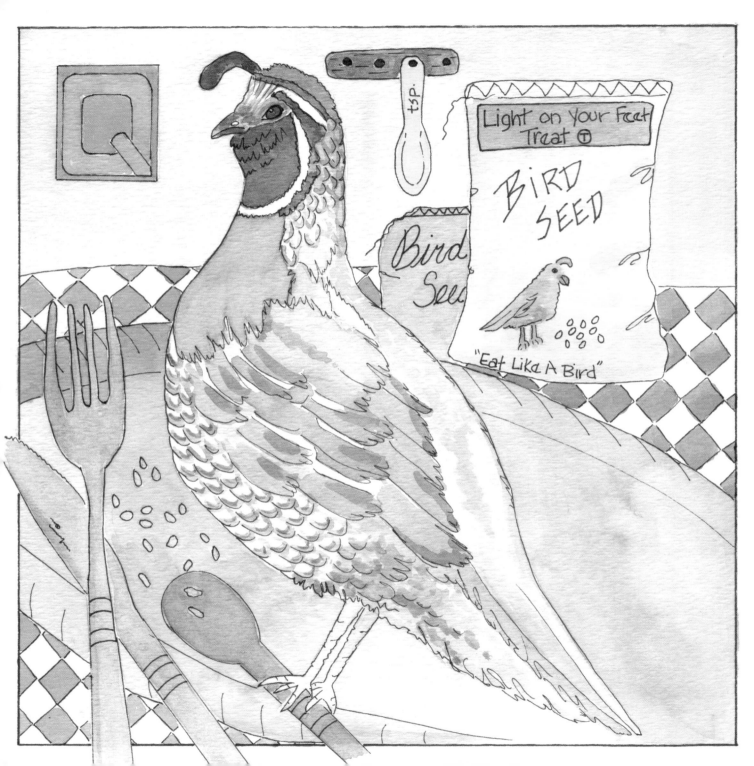

Quail are noted for
eating like birds.

Quantity for them is
too silly for words.

They know if you're careful
and don't overeat

You'll be in great shape and
stay light on your feet.

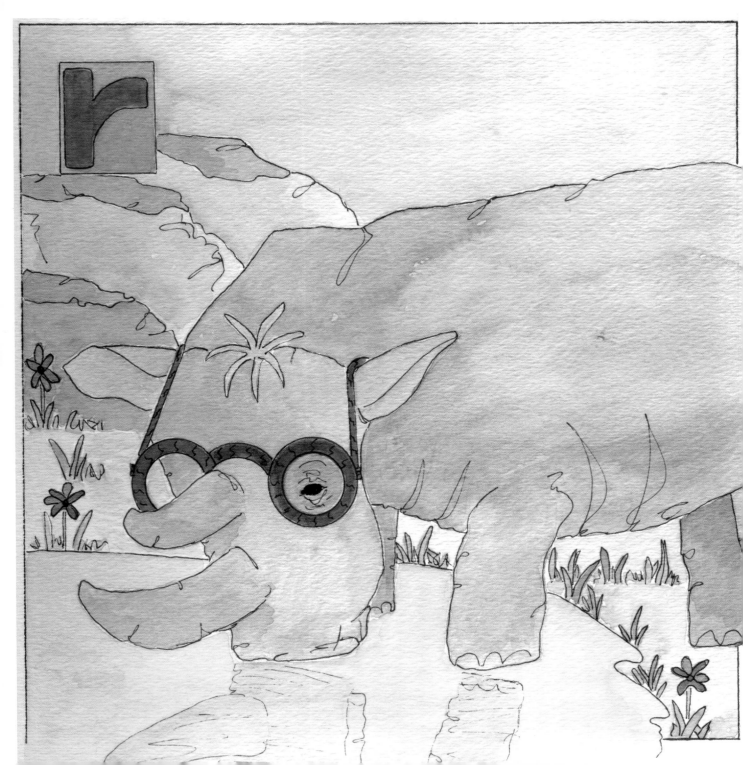

The rhinoceros never looks in
the mirror when alone.

He's aware of thin hair and
his poor muscle tone.

Riboflavin or B-2 would
clear this up fast.

In addition, poor vision would
be a thing of the past.

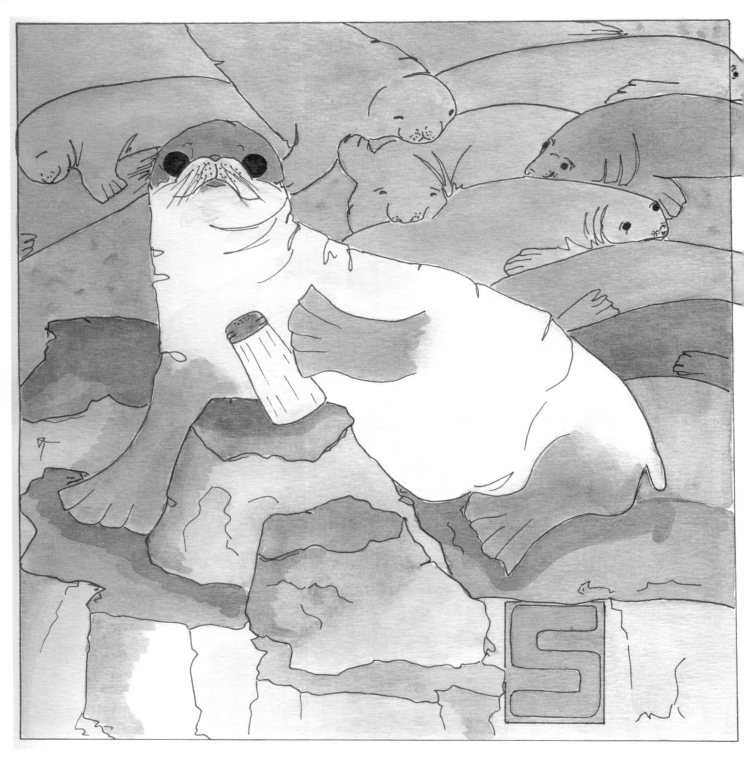

Using sodium and chloride
  (better known as plain salt)

Is a practice that many
  should bring to a halt.

The seal flips his shaker
  away from the table.

This trick keeps him cool and
  his blood pressure stable.

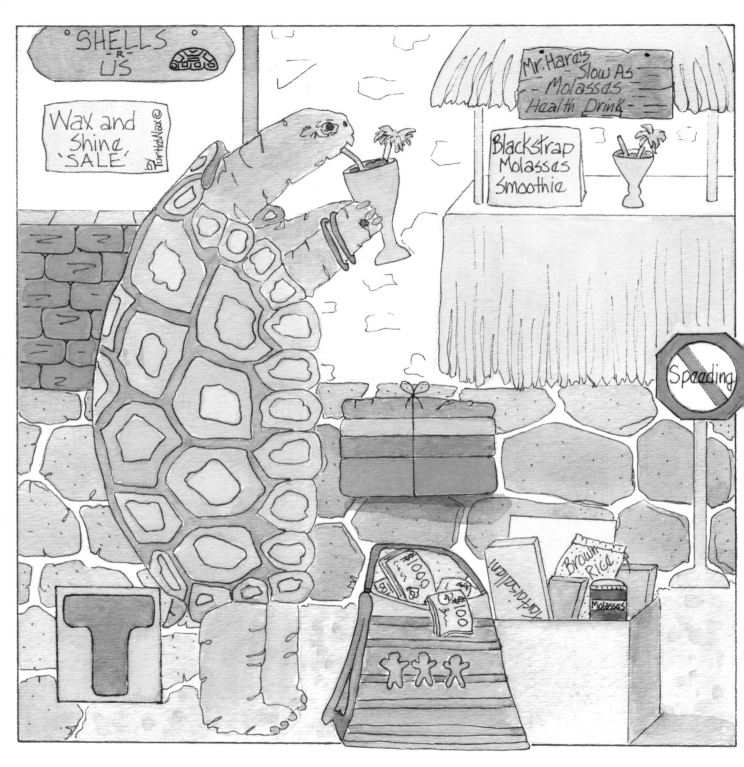

On the turtle's shopping trips
she will pay any price

For blackstrap molasses or her
favorite whole brown rice.

"After all's said and done what's
the use of being wealthy

If I lack thiamine to keep my
nervous system healthy?"

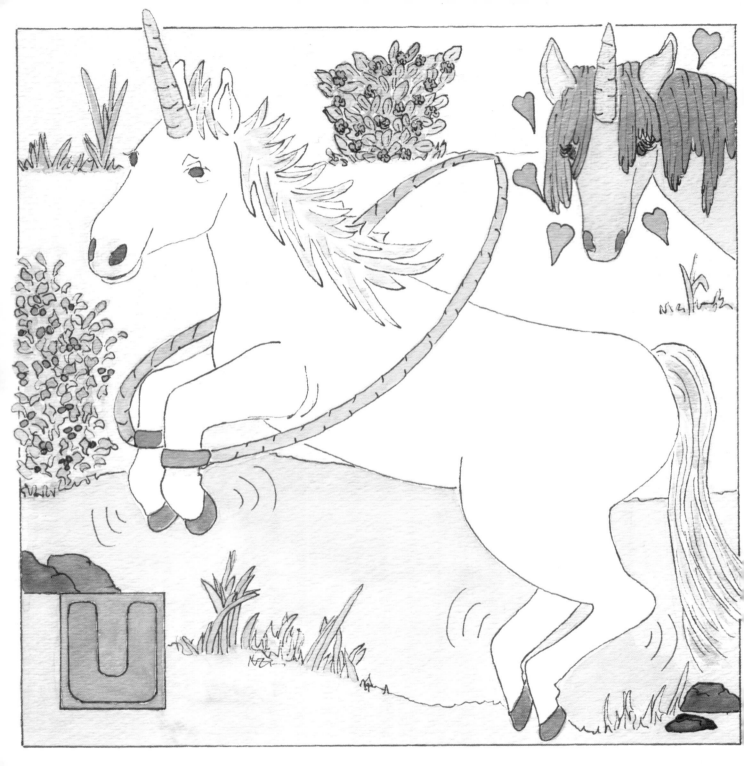

"Skipping a meal gives
me really no hope."

The unicorn mutters
while skipping a rope.

"I'll be undernourished,
run down and feel tired

And by my own friends
ne'er be admired."

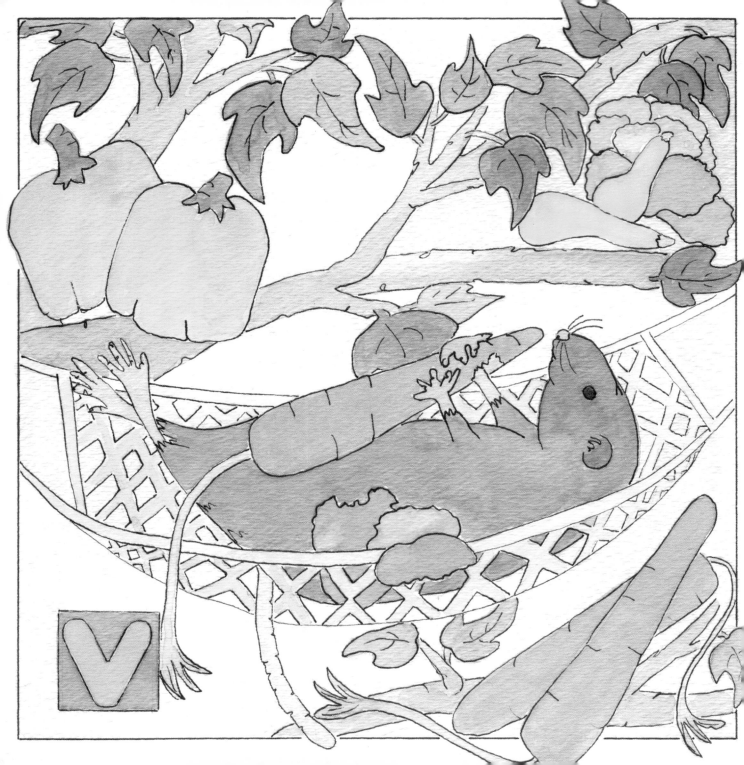

Vegetables do vary for
the vole—a smart fellow,

Who tried many kinds; some
are green, some are yellow.

He has many favorites,
too numerous to mention

Including crisp carrots which
he gnaws to ease tension.

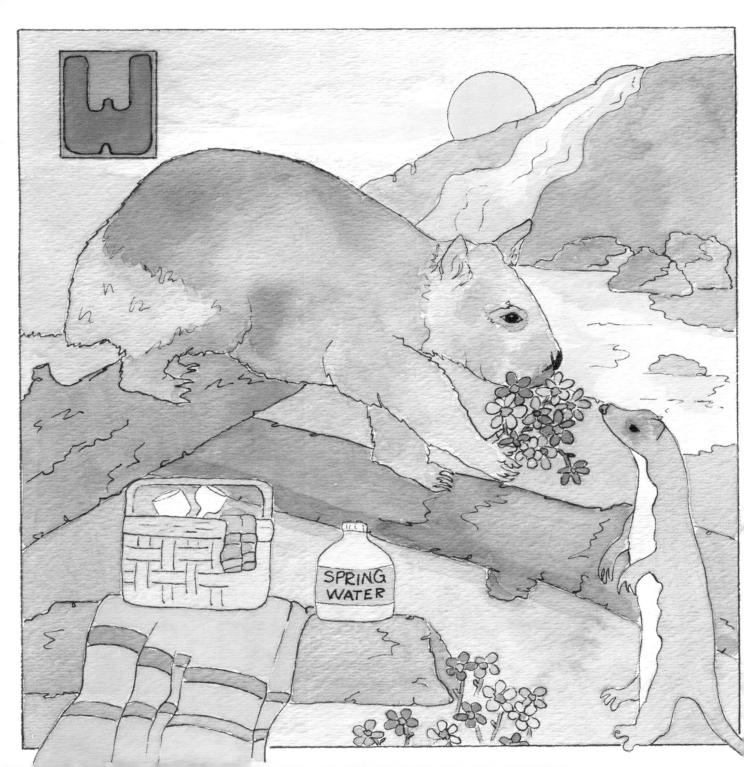

The wise wombat while wooing
the weasel's wee daughter

Took a mighty big sip from
a glass of fresh water.

He did this quite often
as one who does think

That there's no doubt that this
is the world's greatest drink.

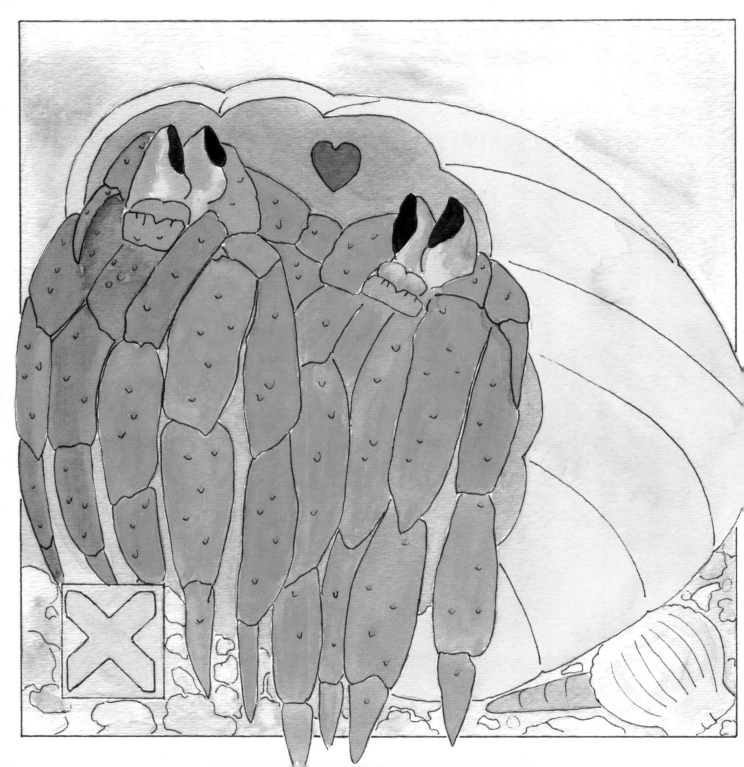

The crab family, Xanthidae,
both Mr. and Mrs.

Know full well the value
of XX's (or kisses).

They feel that love
as well as good diet

Is very important.
Ready to try it?

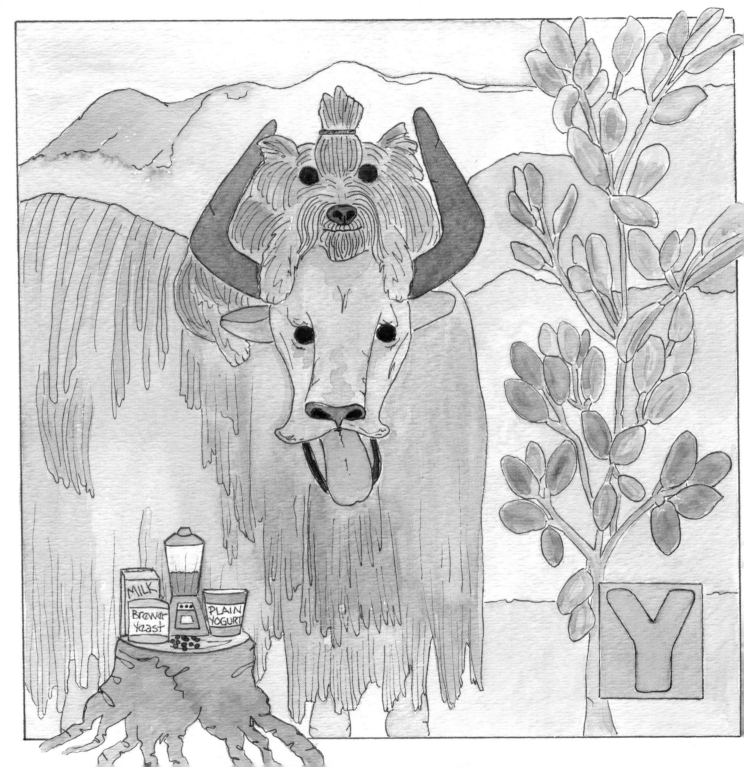

"Why?" asks the Yorkshire terrier so small,

"Is there nothing nutritious with my letter at all?"

"There's yeast and there's yogurt," says the young, yawning yak.

"With both in your diet, good health you'll not lack."

PLAIN YOGURT

BREWER'S YEAST

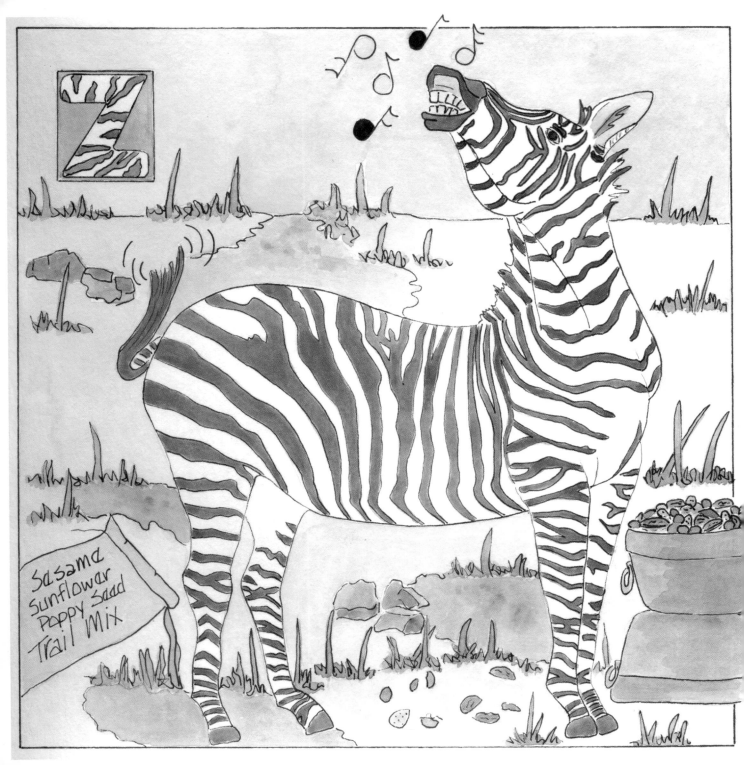

The zebra takes zinc
as part of his feast

By nibbling on nuts, seeds
or plain brewers yeast.

It helps with digestion
and also in healing

And what's more it gives him
a very good feeling.

The Author

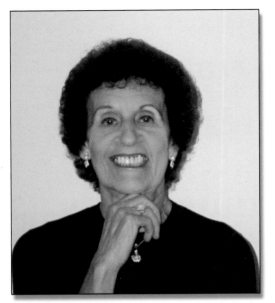

A native Chicagoan, Sallie O'Donnell received her education at the University of Chicago and the University of Illinois. Her teaching career spanned 33 years in both New York City and Orlando, FL. She has written articles on educational topics for the Orlando Sentinel, New Smyrna Beach Observer, Florida English Journal, and a variety of magazines. She lives in New Smyrna Beach, FL with her husband, two bichon frises and two poodles. This is her first children's book.

The Illustrator

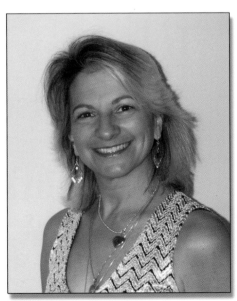

Alea Plumley was born in Drexel Hill, PA and has thirty years experience in a variety of art venues. After attending Philadelphia College of Textiles and Sciences, she applied her talents to murals, graphic design and illustration, watercolor, mosaics, dance, theater and more. She always says, "I am 99% creative energy and 1% logic." She is now living in Palm Bay, FL with friends, fourteen cats, and counting.